Lean and Green Cookbook 2021

Super Tasty, Quick and Easy Wholesome vegetarian recipes That Aiming to Establish a Healthy Lifestyle

Crystal Valdez

Contents

Introduction

What is Lean and Green Diet

Lean and Green diet is basically a weight loss or weight maintenance program that suggests the use of a lean and green meal along with processed food called "fueling." And here is the concept of fueling is organized around the whole Lean and Green Diet:

- The diet says to add nutritional Fuelings to the diet while controlling the overall caloric intake.
- The fueling is actually powdered food, which is mixed with liquid like water and then added to the diet as a part of routine meals.
- Besides consuming these fueling, the dieters are also suggested to exercise 30 minutes daily to lose their weight.
- By trying fueling as a substitute for real food, you can curb the carb and sugar intake and can manage your caloric intake as well.

How much Fuelings to consume, how much food to eat, and what to eat on this dietary regime depends on the type of weight loss plan you are going for. However, on this diet, the overall calorie intake for adults is reduced to 800 to 1000 per day, which lets you lose about 12 lbs. of weight per 12 weeks on average.

Weight-loss Benefits of Lean and Green Diet

Our caloric intake should be around 1000 calories per day in order to initiate weight-loss fat burning in the body. But cutting down your calories just by avoiding food is not the solution. A dieter needs help to maintain his low-caloric intake and meet all the nutritional needs as well. The Lean and Green Diet thus provides a perfect solution- the food Fuelings. A fueling is made specially to keep the calories low and provide all the essential nutrients that are required to carry out the normal metabolic activities in the body. Each fueling is created to have only 100 to 110 calories, which is low enough to keep the daily caloric intake to 1000 calories.

Eating on Lean and Green Diet

The lean and green meal must have the following essential ingredients to keep it healthy and safe:

- **Seafood:**

Seafood is best to have on any weight loss regime because it is free from saturated fats and brings a lot of nutritional value to the table. You can have all types of fishes and seafood on this diet, including halibut, salmon, trout, lobster, tuna, shrimp, crab, and scallops, etc.

- **Meat:**

The lean and green diet only allows 85 percent of lean meat on a diet; whether it is chicken, beef, turkey, lamb, pork, and ground meat, it all has to be lean. Lean meat has lower fat content, which makes it great to keep the caloric intake in control.

- **Eggs:**

Eggs are rich in protein, and they are low in carbs; that's what makes eggs the right for this diet.

- **Soy products:**

In soy products, tofu is the only product that is allowed on the diet because it is processed, and the caloric content is suitable for the lean diet.

- **Fats:**

Not all fats are healthy, and there are a handful of options that you must try on this diet, which includes most of the vegetable olive oil, walnut oil, canola oil, flaxseed oil.

- **Low carb vegetables:**

Focus on all the green veggies for this diet. Except for potatoes, yams, sweet potatoes, yellow squash, and beetroots, you can try every other vegetable on this diet, including cabbage, spinach, cucumbers, etc.

- Sugar-free snacks
- Sugar-free beverages
- Condiments and seasonings

Lean and Green Cookbook 2021

Foods to Avoid

As the Lean and Green diet is restrictive in approach, there is a certain food that is not allowed on this diet. The following food must be avoided.

- All fried foods
- High carb refined grain items
- Saturated fats
- Milk
- All varieties of alcohol
- All sweetened beverages

Vegetarian Recipes

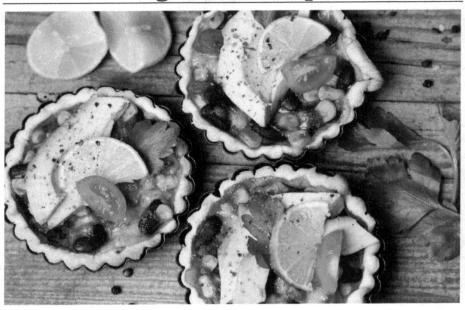

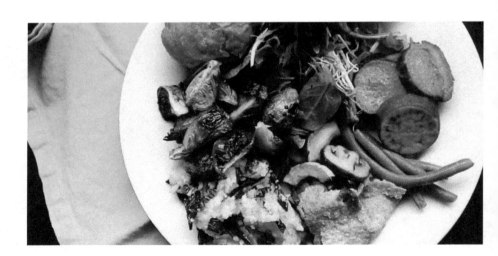

Avocado Toast

Servings: 4
Preparation Time: 15 minutes
Cooking Time: 4 minutes

Ingredients:

- 1 large avocado, peeled, pitted and chopped roughly
- ¼ teaspoon fresh lemon juice
- Salt and ground black pepper, as required
- 4 whole-wheat bread slices
- 4 hard-boiled eggs, peeled and sliced

Instructions:

1. In a bowl, add the avocado and with a fork, mash roughly.
2. Add the lemon juice, salt and black pepper and stir to combine well and Set aside.
3. Heat a nonstick frying pan on medium-high heat and toast the slice for about 2 minutes per side.
4. Repeat with the remaining slices.
5. Spread the avocado mixture over each slice evenly.
6. Top each with egg slices and serve immediately.

Nutritional Information per Serving:

Calories: 206
Fat: 13.9g
Carbohydrates: 14g
Fiber: 4.5g
Sugar: 1.4g
Protein: 9.6g
Sodium: 224mg

Baked Eggs

Servings: 6
Preparation Time: 10 minutes
Cooking Time: 9 minutes

Ingredients:

- 2 cups fresh spinach, chopped finely
- 12 large eggs
- ½ cup heavy cream
- ¾ cup low-fat parmesan cheese, shredded
- Salt and ground black pepper, as required

Instructions:

1. Preheat your oven to 425 degrees F.
2. Grease a 12 cups muffin tin.
3. Divide spinach in each muffin cup.
4. Crack an egg over spinach into each cup and drizzle with heavy cream.
5. Sprinkle with salt and black pepper, followed by Parmesan cheese.
6. Bake for approximately 7-9 minutes or until desired doneness of eggs.
7. Serve immediately.

Nutritional Information per Serving:

Calories: 213
Fat: 16.2g
Carbohydrates: 1.6g
Fiber: 0.2g
Sugar: 0.8g
Protein: 15.6g
Sodium: 370mg

Eggs in Bell Pepper Rings

Servings: 2
Preparation Time: 10 minutes
Cooking Time: 6 minutes

Ingredients:

- 1 bell pepper, seeded and cut into 4 (¼-inch) rings
- 4 eggs
- Salt and ground black pepper, as required
- 1 tablespoon fresh parsley, chopped
- 1 tablespoon fresh chives, chopped

Instructions:

1. Heat a lightly greased nonstick wok over medium heat
2. Place 4 bell pepper rings in the wok and cook for about 2 minutes.
3. Carefully flip the rings.
4. Crack an egg in the middle of each bell pepper ring and sprinkle with salt and black pepper.
5. Cook for about 2-4 minutes or until desired doneness of eggs.
6. Carefully transfer the bell pepper rings ono serving plates and serve with the garnishing of parsley and chives.

Nutritional Information per Serving:

Calories: 139
Fat: 8.9g
Carbohydrates: 3.6g
Fiber: 1.1g
Sugar: 2.2g
Protein: 11.7g
Sodium: 327mg

Eggs in Avocado Halves

Servings: 2
Preparation Time: 10 minutes
Cooking Time: 15 minutes

Ingredients:

- 1 avocado, halved and pitted
- 2 eggs
- Salt and ground black pepper, as required
- ¼ cup cherry tomatoes, halved
- 2 cups fresh baby spinach

Instructions:

1. Preheat your oven to 425 degrees F.
2. Carefully remove about 2 tablespoons of flesh from each avocado half.
3. Place avocado halves into a small baking dish.
4. Carefully crack an egg in each avocado half and sprinkle with salt and black pepper.
5. Bake for approximately 15 minutes or until desired doneness of the eggs.
6. Arrange 1 avocado half onto each serving plate and serve alongside the cherry tomatoes and spinach.

Nutritional Information per Serving:

Calories: 247
Fat: 21.1g
Carbohydrates: 9.6g
Fiber: 6.6g
Sugar: 1.5g
Protein: 8.2g
Sodium: 169mg

Broccoli Waffles

Servings: 2
Preparation Time: 10 minutes
Cooking Time: 8 minutes

Ingredients:

- 1/3 cup broccoli, chopped finely
- ¼ cup low-fat cheddar cheese, shredded
- 1 egg
- ½ teaspoon garlic powder
- ½ teaspoon dried onion, minced
- Salt and ground black pepper, as required

Instructions:

1. Preheat a mini waffle iron and then grease it.
2. In a medium bowl, place all ingredients and mix until well combined.
3. Place ½ of the mixture into preheated waffle iron and cook for about 3-4 minutes or until golden brown.
4. Repeat with the remaining mixture.
5. Serve warm.

Nutritional Information per Serving:

Calories: 96
Fat: 6.9g
Carbohydrates: 2g
Fiber: 0.5g
Sugar: 0.7g
Protein: 6.8g
Sodium: 97mg

Cheesy Spinach Waffles

Servings: 4
Preparation Time: 10 minutes
Cooking Time: 20 minutes

Ingredients:

- 1 large egg, beaten
- 1 cup ricotta cheese, crumbled
- ½ cup part-skim mozzarella cheese, shredded
- ¼ cup low-fat Parmesan cheese, grated
- 4 ounces frozen spinach, thawed and squeezed dry
- 1 garlic clove, minced
- Salt and ground black pepper, as required

Instructions:

1. Preheat a mini waffle iron and then grease it.
2. In a bowl, add all the ingredients and beat until well combined.
3. Place ¼ of the mixture into preheated waffle iron and cook for about 4-5 minutes or until golden brown.
4. Repeat with the remaining mixture.
5. Serve warm.

Nutritional Information per Serving:

Calories: 138
Fat: 8.1g
Carbohydrates: 4.8g
Fiber: 0.6g
Sugar: 0.4g
Protein: 11.7g
Sodium: 273mg

Kale Scramble

Servings: 2
Preparation Time: 10 minutes
Cooking Time: 6 minutes

Ingredients:

- 4 eggs
- 1/8 teaspoon ground turmeric
- 1/8 teaspoon red pepper flakes, crushed
- Salt and ground black pepper, as required
- 1 tablespoon water
- 2 teaspoons olive oil
- 1 cup fresh kale, tough ribs removed and chopped

Instructions:

1. In a bowl, add the eggs, turmeric, red pepper flakes, salt, black pepper and water and with a whisk, beat until foamy.
2. In a wok, heat the oil over medium heat
3. Add the egg mixture and stir to combine.
4. Immediately reduce the heat to medium-low and cook for about 1-2 minutes, stirring frequently.
5. Stir in the kale and cook for about 3-4 minutes, stirring frequently.
6. Remove from the heat and serve immediately.

Nutritional Information per Serving:

Calories: 183
Fat: 13.4g
Carbohydrates: 4.3g
Fiber: 0.5g
Sugar: 0.7g
Protein: 12.1g
Sodium: 216mg

Tomato & Egg Scramble

Servings: 2
Preparation Time: 10 minutes
Cooking Time: 5 minutes

Ingredients:

- 4 eggs
- ¼ teaspoon red pepper flakes, crushed
- Salt and ground black pepper, as required
- ¼ cup fresh basil, chopped
- ½ cup tomatoes, chopped
- 1 tablespoon olive oil

Instructions:

1. In a large bowl, add eggs, red pepper flakes, salt and black pepper and beat well.
2. Add the basil and tomatoes and stir to combine.
3. In a large non-stick wok, heat the oil over medium-high heat.
4. Add the egg mixture and cook for about 3-5 minutes, stirring continuously.
5. Serve immediately.

Nutritional Information per Serving:

Calories: 195
Fat: 15.9g
Carbohydrates: 2.6g
Fiber: 0.7g
Sugar: 1.9g
Protein: 11.6g
Sodium: 203mg

Tofu & Spinach Scramble

Servings: 2
Preparation Time: 10 minutes
Cooking Time: 8 minutes

Ingredients:

- 1 tablespoon olive oil
- 1 garlic clove, minced
- ¼ pound medium-firm tofu, drained, pressed and crumbled
- 1/3 cup low-sodium vegetable broth
- 2¾ cups fresh baby spinach
- 2 teaspoons low-sodium soy sauce
- 1 teaspoon ground turmeric
- 1 teaspoon fresh lemon juice

Instructions:

1. In a frying pan, heat the olive oil over medium-high heat and sauté the garlic for about 1 minute
2. Add the tofu and cook for about 2-3 minutes, slowly adding the broth.
3. Add the spinach, soy sauce and turmeric and stir fry for about 3-4 minutes or until all the liquid is absorbed
4. Stir in the lemon juice and remove from the heat.
5. Serve immediately.

Nutritional Information per Serving:

Calories: 134
Fat: 10.1g
Carbohydrates: 5.8g
Fiber: 2.7g
Sugar: 1.3g
Protein: 8.5g
Sodium: 497mg

Tofu & Veggie Scramble

Servings: 2
Preparation Time: 15 minutes
Cooking Time: 15 minutes

Ingredients:

- ½ tablespoon olive oil
- 1 small onion, chopped finely
- 1 small red bell pepper, seeded and chopped finely
- 1 cup cherry tomatoes, chopped finely
- 1½ cups firm tofu, crumbled and chopped
- Pinch of cayenne pepper
- Pinch of ground turmeric
- Sea salt, as required

Instructions:

1. In a wok, heat oil over medium heat and sauté the onion and bell pepper for about 4-5 minutes.
2. Add the tomatoes and cook for about 1-2 minutes.
3. Add the tofu, turmeric, cayenne pepper and salt and cook for about 6-8 minutes.
4. Serve hot.

Nutritional Information per Serving:

Calories: 201
Fat: 11.7g
Carbohydrates: 11g
Fiber: 4.2g
Sugar: 5.9g
Protein: 17g
Sodium: 147mg

Apple Omelet

Servings: 1
Preparation Time: 10 minutes
Cooking Time: 9 minutes

Ingredients:

- 2 teaspoons olive oil, divided
- ½ of large green apple, cored and sliced thinly
- ¼ teaspoon ground cinnamon
- 1/8 teaspoon ground nutmeg
- 2 large eggs
- 1/8 teaspoon vanilla extract
- Pinch of salt

Instructions:

1. In a nonstick frying pan, heat 1 teaspoon of oil over medium-low heat
2. Add apple slices and sprinkle with nutmeg and cinnamon.
3. Cook for about 4-5 minutes, turning once halfway through.
4. Meanwhile, in a bowl, add eggs, vanilla extract and salt and beat until fluffy.
5. Add the remaining oil in the pan and let it heat completely.
6. Place the egg mixture over apple slices evenly and cook for about 3-4 minutes or until desired doneness.
7. Carefully turn the pan over a serving plate and immediately fold the omelet
8. Serve hot.

Nutritional Information per Serving:

Calories: 258
Fat: 19.5g
Carbohydrates: 9g
Fiber: 1.2g
Sugar: 7g

Protein: 12.8g
Sodium: 295mg

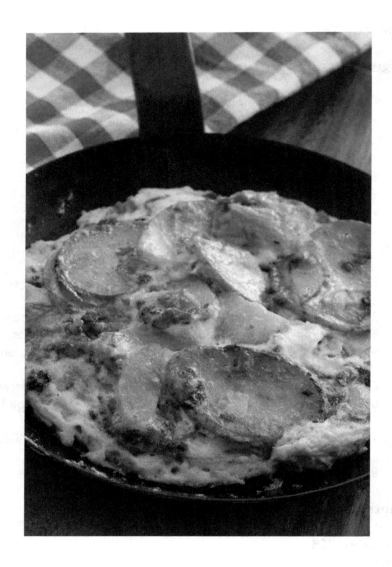

Mushroom & Tomato Omelet

Servings: 2
Preparation Time: 15 minutes
Cooking Time: 36 minutes

Ingredients:

- 2 poblano peppers
- Olive oil cooking spray
- 1 small tomato
- ½ teaspoon dried oregano
- ½ teaspoon chicken bouillon seasoning
- 4 eggs, separated
- 2 tablespoons sour cream
- ½ cup fresh white mushrooms, sliced
- 2/3 cup part-skim mozzarella cheese, shredded and divided

Instructions:

1. Preheat your oven to broiler.
2. Line a baking sheet with a piece of foil.
3. Spray the poblano peppers with cooking spray lightly.
4. Arrange the peppers onto the prepared baking sheet in a single layer and broil for about 5-10 minutes per side or until skin becomes dark ad blistered.
5. Remove from the oven and set aside to cool.
6. After cooking, remove the stems, skin and seeds from peppers and then cut each into thin strips.
7. Meanwhile, for sauce: with a knife, make 2 small slits in a crisscross pattern on the top of tomato.
8. In a microwave-safe plate, place the tomato and microwave on High for about 2-3 minutes.
9. In a blender, add the tomato, oregano and chicken bouillon seasoning and pulse until smooth.
10. Transfer the sauce into a bowl and set aside.
11. In a bowl, add the egg yolks and sour cream and beat until well combined.

12. In a clean glass bowl, add egg whites and with an electric mixer, beat until soft peaks form
13. Gently gold the egg yolk mixture into whipped egg whites
14. Heat a lightly greased wok over medium-low heat and cook half of the egg mixture cook for about 3-5 minutes or until bottom is set
15. Place half of the mushrooms and pepper strips over one half of omelet and sprinkle with half of the cheese
16. Cover the wok and cook for about 2-3 minutes
17. Uncover the wok and fold in the omelet
18. Transfer the omelet onto a plate
19. Repeat with the remaining egg mixture, mushrooms, pepper strips and cheese.
20. Top each omelet with sauce and serve.

Nutritional Information per Serving:

Calories: 209
Fat: 13.2g
Carbohydrates: 8.4g
Fiber: 1.6g
Sugar: 4.5g
Protein: 16g
Sodium: 193mg

Veggie Omelet

Servings: 4
Preparation Time: 10 minutes
Cooking Time: 25 minutes

Ingredients:

- 6 large eggs
- ½ cup unsweetened almond milk
- Salt and ground black pepper, as required
- ½ of onion, chopped
- ¼ cup bell pepper, seeded and chopped
- ¼ cup fresh mushrooms, sliced
- 1 tablespoon chives, minced

Instructions:

1. Preheat your oven to 350 degrees F.
2. Lightly grease a pie dish.
3. In a bowl, add eggs, almond milk, salt and black pepper and beat until well combined.
4. In a separate bowl, mix together onion, bell pepper and mushrooms.
5. Place the egg mixture into the prepared pie dish evenly and top with vegetable mixture.
6. Sprinkle with chives evenly.
7. Bake for approximately 20-25 minutes.
8. Remove the pie dish from oven and set aside for about 5 minutes.
9. Cut into 4 portions and serve immediately.

Nutritional Information per Serving:

Calories: 121
Fat: 8g
Carbohydrates: 2.8g
Fiber: 0.6g
Sugar: 0.1g
Protein: 10.1g
Sodium: 167mg

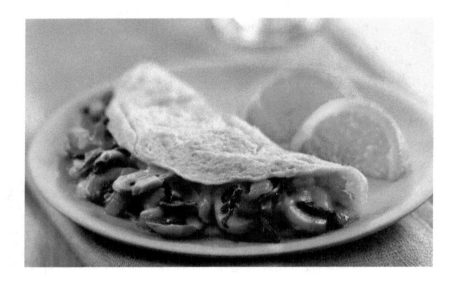

Veggies Quiche

Servings: 4
Preparation Time: 15 minutes
Cooking Time: 25 minutes

Ingredients:

- 6 large eggs
- Salt and ground black pepper, as required
- ½ cup unsweetened almond milk
- ½ of onion, chopped
- ¼ cup fresh mushrooms, cut into slices
- ¼ cup red bell pepper, seeded and diced
- 1 tablespoon fresh chives, minced

Instructions:

1. Preheat your oven to 350 degrees F.
2. Lightly grease a pie dish.
3. In a bowl, add the eggs, salt, black pepper and coconut oil and beat until well combined.
4. In another bowl, mix together the onion, bell pepper and mushrooms.
5. Transfer the egg mixture into the prepared pie dish evenly.
6. Top with the vegetable mixture evenly.
7. Sprinkle with chives evenly.
8. Bake for approximately 20-25 minutes.
9. Remove the pie dish from oven and set aside for about 5 minutes.
10. Cut into equal-sized wedges and serve.

Nutritional Information per Serving:

Calories: 121
Fat: 8g
Carbohydrates: 2.9g
Fiber: 0.6g
Sugar: 1.6g
Protein: 10g
Sodium: 187mg

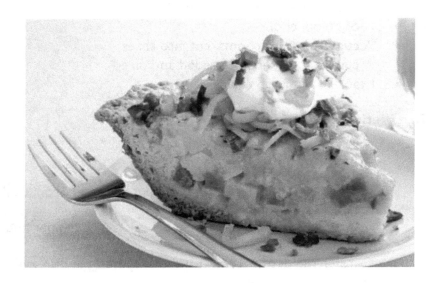

Zucchini & Carrot Quiche

Servings: 3
Preparation Time: 10 minutes
Cooking Time: 40 minutes

Ingredients:

- 5 eggs
- Salt and ground black pepper, as required
- 1 carrot, peeled and grated
- 1 small zucchini, shredded

Instructions:

1. Preheat your oven to 350 degrees F.
2. Lightly grease a small baking dish.
3. In a large bowl, add eggs, salt and black pepper and beat well
4. Add the carrot and zucchini and stir to combine
5. Transfer the mixture into the prepared baking dish evenly
6. Bake for approximately 40 minutes.
7. Remove the baking dish from oven and set aside for about 5 minutes.
8. Cut into equal-sized wedges and serve.

Nutritional Information per Serving:

Calories: 119
Fat: 7.4g
Carbohydrates: 3.9g
Fiber: 0.9g
Sugar: 2.2g
Protein: 9.9g
Sodium: 171mg

Green Veggies Quiche

Servings: 4
Preparation Time: 15 minutes
Cooking Time: 20 minutes

Ingredients:

- 6 eggs
- ½ cup unsweetened almond milk
- Salt and ground black pepper, as required
- 2 cups fresh baby spinach, chopped
- ½ cup green bell pepper, seeded and chopped
- 1 scallion, chopped
- ¼ cup fresh cilantro, chopped
- 1 tablespoon fresh chives, minced
- 3 tablespoons part-skim mozzarella cheese, grated

Instructions:

1. Preheat your oven to 400 degrees F.
2. Lightly grease a pie dish
3. In a large bowl, add the eggs, almond milk, salt and black pepper and beat until well combined. Set aside.
4. In another bowl, add the vegetables and herbs and mix well.
5. In the bottom of the prepared pie dish, place the veggie mixture evenly and top with the egg mixture.
6. Bake for approximately 20 minutes or until a wooden skewer inserted in the center comes out clean.
7. Remove from the oven and immediately sprinkle with the Parmesan cheese.
8. Set aside for about 5 minutes before slicing.
9. Cut into desired sized wedges and serve.

Nutritional Information per Serving:

Calories: 176
Fat: 4.1g
Carbohydrates: 5g
Fiber: 0.9g
Sugar: 4g
Protein: 15.4g
Sodium: 296mg

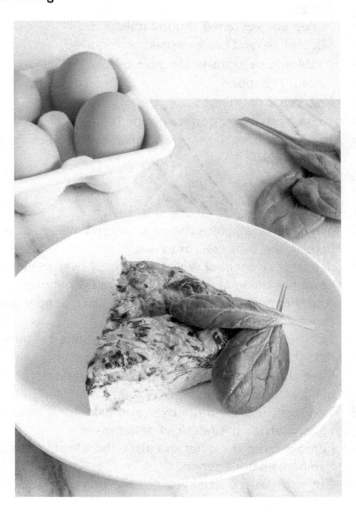

Kale & Mushroom Frittata

Servings: 5
Preparation Time: 15 minutes
Cooking Time: 30 minutes

Ingredients:

- 8 eggs
- ½ cup unsweetened almond milk
- Salt and ground black pepper, as required
- 1 tablespoon extra-virgin olive oil
- 1 onion, chopped
- 1 garlic clove, minced
- 1 cup fresh mushrooms, chopped
- 1 ½ cups fresh kale, tough ribs removed and chopped

Instructions:

1. Preheat your oven to 350 degrees F.
2. In a large bowl, place the eggs, almond milk, salt and black pepper and beat well. Set aside.
3. In a large ovenproof wok, heat the oil over medium heat and sauté the onion and garlic for about 3-4 minutes.
4. Add the mushrooms, kale, salt and black pepper and cook for about 8-10 minutes.
5. Stir in the mushrooms and cook for about 3-4 minutes.
6. Add the kale and cook for about 5 minutes.
7. Place the egg mixture on top evenly and cook for about 4 minutes, without stirring.
8. Transfer the wok in the oven and Bake for approximately 12-15 minutes or until desired doneness.
9. Remove from the oven and place the frittata side for about 3-5 minutes before serving.
10. Cut into desired sized wedges and serve.

Nutritional Information per Serving:

Calories: 151
Fat: 10.2g
Carbohydrates: 5.6g
Fiber: 1g
Sugar: 1.7g
Protein: 10.3g
Sodium: 158mg

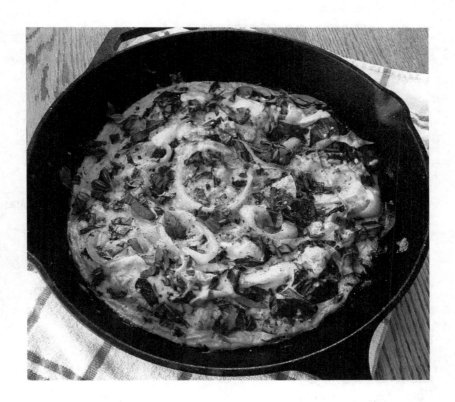

Kale & Bell Pepper Frittata

Servings: 3
Preparation Time: 10 minutes
Cooking Time: 17 minutes

Ingredients:

- 6 eggs
- Salt, as required
- I tablespoon olive oil
- ½ teaspoon ground turmeric
- I small red bell pepper, seeded and chopped
- I cup fresh kale, trimmed and chopped
- ¼ cup fresh chives, chopped

Instructions:

1. In a bowl, add the eggs and salt and beat well. Set aside.
2. In a cast-iron wok, heat the oil over medium-low heat and sprinkle with turmeric.
3. Immediately stir in the bell pepper and kale and sauté for about 2 minutes.
4. Place the beaten eggs over bell pepper mixture evenly and immediately reduce the heat to low.
5. Cover the wok and cook for about 10-15 minutes.
6. Remove from the heat and set aside for about 5 minutes.
7. Cut into equal-sized wedges and serve.

Nutritional Information per Serving:

Calories: 192
Fat: 13.6g
Carbohydrates: 6.4g
Fiber: Ig
Sugar: 2.8g
Protein: 12.3g
Sodium: 185mg

Bell Pepper Frittata

Servings: 6
Preparation Time: 15 minutes
Cooking Time: 10 minutes

Ingredients:

- 8 eggs
- 1 tablespoon fresh cilantro, chopped
- 1 tablespoon fresh basil, chopped
- ¼ teaspoon red pepper flakes, crushed
- Salt and ground black pepper, as required
- 2 tablespoons olive oil
- 1 bunch scallions, chopped
- 1 cup bell pepper, seeded and sliced thinly
- ½ cup goat cheese, crumbled

Instructions:

1. Preheat the broiler of oven.
2. Arrange a rack in upper third of the oven.
3. In a bowl, add the eggs, fresh herbs, red pepper flakes, salt and black pepper and beat well.
4. In an ovenproof wok, heat the oil over medium heat and sauté the scallion and bell pepper for about 1 minute.
5. Add the egg mixture over bell pepper mixture evenly and lift the edges to let the egg mixture flow underneath and cook for about 2-3 minutes.
6. Place the cheese on top in the form of dots.
7. Now, transfer the wok under broiler and broil for about 2-3 minutes.
8. Remove from the oven and set aside for about 5 minutes before serving.
9. Cut the frittata into desired sized slices and serve.

Nutritional Information per Serving:

Calories: 193
Fat: 15.2g
Carbohydrates: 3.2g
Fiber: 0.5g
Sugar: 1.6g
Protein: 11.7g
Sodium: 284mg

Broccoli Frittata

Servings: 6
Preparation Time: 15 minutes
Cooking Time: 13 minutes

Ingredients:

- 8 eggs
- 1 tablespoon fresh cilantro, chopped
- 1 tablespoon fresh basil, chopped
- ¼ teaspoon red pepper flakes, crushed
- Salt and ground black pepper, as required
- 2 tablespoons olive oil
- 1 bunch scallions, chopped
- 1 cup broccoli, chopped finely
- ½ cup goat cheese, crumbled

Instructions:

1. Preheat the broiler of oven.
2. Arrange a rack in upper third of oven.
3. In a bowl, add eggs, fresh herbs, red pepper flakes, salt and black pepper and beat well.
4. In an ovenproof wok, heat the oil over medium heat and sauté scallion and broccoli for about 1-2 minutes.
5. Add the egg mixture over the broccoli mixture evenly and lift the edges to let the egg mixture flow underneath.
6. Cook for about 2-3 minutes.
7. Place the cheese on top in the form of dots.
8. Now, transfer the wok under broiler and broil for about 2-3 minutes.
9. Remove the wok from oven and set aside for about 5 minutes.
10. Cut the frittata into desired size slices and serve.

Nutritional Information per Serving:

Calories: 192
Fat: 15.3g
Carbohydrates: 2.8g
Fiber: 0.6g
Sugar: 0.9g
Protein: 12g
Sodium: 316mg

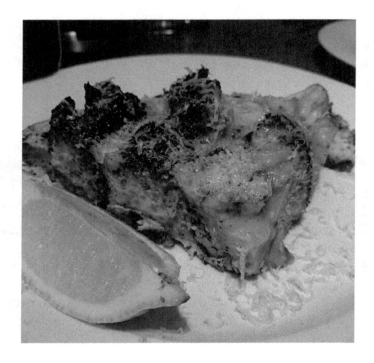

Zucchini Frittata

Servings: 6
Preparation Time: 15 minutes
Cooking Time: 20 minutes

Ingredients:

- 2 tablespoons unsweetened almond milk
- 8 eggs
- Freshly ground black pepper, as required
- 1 tablespoon olive oil
- 1 garlic clove, minced
- 2 medium zucchinis, cut into ¼-inch thick round slices
- ½ cup goat cheese, crumbled

Instructions:

1. Preheat your oven to 350 degrees F.
2. In a bowl, add the almond milk, eggs and black pepper and black pepper and beat well.
3. In an ovenproof wok, heat the oil over medium heat and sauté the garlic for about 1 minute.
4. Stir in the zucchini and cook for about 5 minutes.
5. Add the egg mixture and stir for about 1 minute.
6. Sprinkle the cheese on top evenly.
7. Immediately transfer the wok into the oven.
8. Bake for approximately 12 minutes or until eggs become set.
9. Remove from oven and set aside to cool for about 5 minutes.
10. Cut into desired sized wedges and serve.

Nutritional Information per Serving:

Calories: 149
Fat: 11g
Carbohydrates: 3.4g
Fiber: 0.8g
Sugar: 2.1g
Protein: 10g
Sodium: 274mg

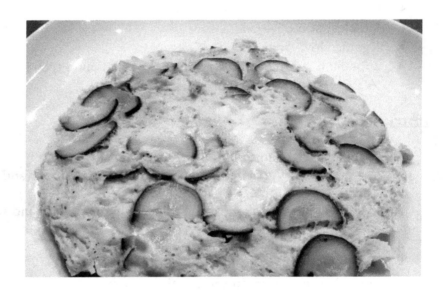

Eggs with Spinach

Servings: 2
Preparation Time: 10 minutes
Cooking Time: 22 minutes

Ingredients:

- 6 cups fresh baby spinach
- 2-3 tablespoons water
- 4 eggs
- Salt and ground black pepper, as required
- 2-3 tablespoons feta cheese, crumbled

Instructions:

1. Preheat your oven to 400 degrees F.
2. Lightly grease 2 small baking dishes.
3. In a large frying pan, add spinach and water over medium heat and cook for about 3-4 minutes.
4. Remove the frying pan from heat and drain the excess water completely.
5. Divide the spinach into prepared baking dishes evenly.
6. Carefully crack 2 eggs in each baking dish over spinach.
7. Sprinkle with salt and black pepper and top with feta cheese evenly.
8. Arrange the baking dishes onto a large cookie sheet.
9. Bake for approximately 15-18 minutes.
10. Serve warm.

Nutritional Information per Serving:

Calories: 171
Fat: 11.1g
Carbohydrates: 4.3g
Fiber: 2g
Sugar: 1.4g
Protein: 15g
Sodium: 377mg

Eggs with Kale & Tomatoes

Servings: 4
Preparation Time: 15 minutes
Cooking Time: 25 minutes

Ingredients:

- 2 tablespoons olive oil
- 1 yellow onion, chopped
- 2 garlic cloves, minced
- 1 cup tomatoes, chopped
- ½ pound fresh kale, tough ribs removed and chopped
- 1 teaspoon ground cumin
- ¼ teaspoon red pepper flakes, crushed
- Salt and ground black pepper, as required
- 4 eggs
- 2 tablespoons fresh parsley, chopped

Instructions:

1. In a large nonstick wok, heat the olive oil over medium heat and sauté the onion for about 4-5 minutes.
2. Add in the garlic and sauté for about 1 minute.
3. Add the tomatoes, spices, salt and black pepper and cook for about 2-3 minutes, stirring frequently.
4. Add in the kale and cook for about 4-5 minutes.
5. Carefully crack eggs on top of kale mixture.
6. With the lid, cover the wok and cook for about 10 minutes or until desired doneness of eggs.
7. Serve hot with the garnishing of parsley.

Nutritional Information per Serving:

Calories: 175
Fat: 11.7g
Carbohydrates: 11g
Fiber: 2.2g
Sugar: 2.8g
Protein: 8.2g
Sodium: 130mg

Eggs with Veggies

Servings: 4
Preparation Time: 10 minutes
Cooking Time: 15 minutes

Ingredients:

- 2 tablespoons olive oil, divided
- ¾ pound zucchini, quartered and sliced thinly
- 1 red bell pepper, seeded and chopped
- 1 medium onion, chopped
- 1 teaspoon fresh rosemary, chopped finely
- Salt and ground black pepper, as required
- 4 large eggs

Instructions:

1. In a large wok, heat 1 tablespoon of oil over medium-high heat and sauté the zucchini, bell pepper and onion for about 5-8 minutes.
2. Add the rosemary, salt and black pepper and stir to combine.
3. With a wooden spoon, make a large well in the center of wok by moving the veggie mixture towards the sides.
4. Reduce the heat to medium and pour the remaining oil in the well.
5. Carefully crack the eggs in the well and sprinkle the eggs with salt and black pepper.
6. Cook for about 1-2 minutes.
7. Cover the wok and cook for about 1-2 minutes more.
8. For serving, carefully scoop the veggie mixture onto 4 serving plates.
9. Top each serving with an egg and serve.

Nutritional Information per Serving:

Calories: 171
Fat: 11.1g
Carbohydrates: 4.3g
Fiber: 2g
Sugar: 1.4g
Protein: 15g
Sodium: 377mg

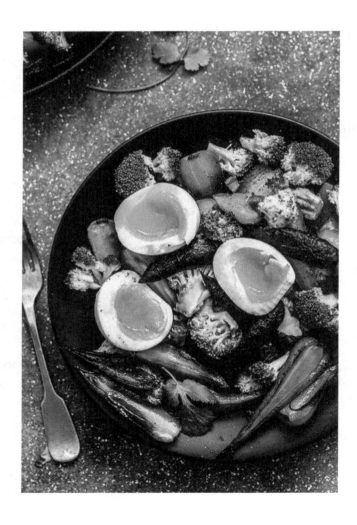

Tofu & Mushroom Muffins

Servings: 6
Preparation Time: 15 minutes
Cooking Time: 30 minutes

Ingredients:

- 2 teaspoons olive oil, divided
- 1 ½ cups fresh mushrooms, chopped
- 1 scallion, chopped
- 1 teaspoon garlic, minced
- 1 teaspoon fresh rosemary, minced
- Freshly ground black pepper, as required
- 1 (12.3-ounce) package lite firm silken tofu, drained
- ¼ cup unsweetened almond milk
- 2 tablespoons nutritional yeast
- 1 tablespoon arrowroot starch
- ¼ teaspoon ground turmeric

Instructions:

1. Preheat your oven to 375 degrees F.
2. Grease a 12 cups muffin tin.
3. In a nonstick wok, heat 1 teaspoon of oil over medium heat and sauté scallion and garlic for about 1 minute.
4. Add mushrooms and sauté for about 5-7 minutes.
5. Stir in the rosemary and black pepper and remove from the heat.
6. Set aside to cool slightly.
7. In a food processor, add tofu and remaining ingredients and pulse until smooth.
8. Transfer the tofu mixture into a large bowl
9. Fold in mushroom mixture.
10. Transfer the mixture into prepared muffin cups evenly.
11. Bake for approximately 20-22 minutes or until a toothpick inserted in the center comes out clean.
12. Remove the muffin pan from the oven and place onto a wire rack to cool for about 10 minutes.
13. Carefully invert the muffins onto the wire rack and serve warm.

Nutritional Information per Serving:

Calories: 70
Fat: 3.6g
Carbohydrates: 4.3g
Fiber: 9.8g
Sugar: 1.3g
Protein: 55.7g
Sodium: 32mg

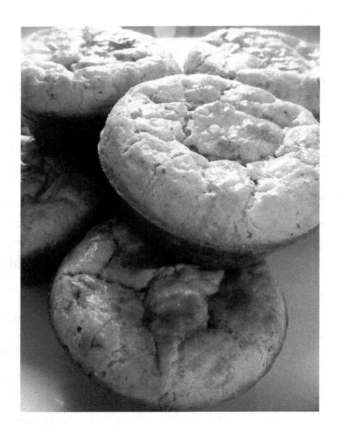

Fruit Salad

Servings: 4
Preparation Time: 15 minutes

Ingredients:

For Salad

- 4 cups fresh baby arugula
- 1 cup fresh strawberries, hulled and sliced
- 2 oranges, peeled and segmented

For Dressing

- 2 tablespoons fresh lemon juice
- 2-3 drops liquid stevia
- 2 teaspoons extra-virgin olive oil
- Salt and ground black pepper, as required

Instructions:

1. **For Salad**: in a salad bowl, place all ingredients and mix.
2. **For Dressing**: place all ingredients in another bowl and beat until well combined.
3. Place dressing on top of salad and toss to coat well.
4. Serve immediately.

Nutritional Information per Serving:

Calories: 82
Fat: 2.7g
Carbohydrates: 13g
Fiber: 3g
Sugar: 10g
Protein: 1.7g
Sodium: 63mg

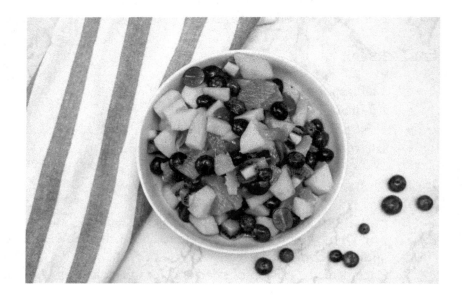

Strawberry, Orange & Rocket Salad

Servings: 4
Preparation Time: 15 minutes

Ingredients:

For Salad:

- 6 cups fresh rocket
- 1 ½ cups fresh strawberries, hulled and sliced
- 2 oranges, peeled and segmented

For Dressing:

- 2 tablespoons fresh lemon juice
- 1 tablespoon raw honey
- 2 teaspoons extra-virgin olive oil
- 1 teaspoon Dijon mustard
- Salt and ground black pepper, as required

Instructions:

1. **For Salad**: in a salad bowl, place all ingredients and mix.
2. **For Dressing**: place all ingredients in another bowl and beat until well combined.
3. Place dressing on top of salad and toss to coat well.
4. Serve immediately.

Nutritional Information per Serving:

Calories: 107
Fat: 2.9g
Carbohydrates: 17g
Fiber: 3.9g
Sugar: 16g
Protein: 2.1g
Sodium: 63mg

Strawberry & Asparagus Salad

Servings: 8
Preparation Time: 15 minutes
Cooking Time: 5 minutes

Ingredients:

- 2 pounds fresh asparagus, trimmed and sliced
- 3 cups fresh strawberries, hulled and sliced
- ¼ cup extra-virgin olive oil
- ¼ cup balsamic vinegar
- 2 tablespoons maple syrup
- Salt and ground black pepper, as required

Instructions:

1. In a pan of water, add the asparagus over medium-high heat and bring to a boil.
2. Boil the asparagus for about 2-3 minutes or until al dente.
3. Drain the asparagus and immediately transfer into a bowl of ice water to cool completely.
4. Drain the asparagus and pat dry with paper towels.
5. In a large bowl, add the asparagus and strawberries and mix.
6. In a small bowl, add the olive oil, vinegar, honey, salt and black pepper and beat until well blended.
7. Place the dressing over the asparagus strawberry mixture and gently toss to coat.
8. Refrigerate for about 1 hour before serving.

Nutritional Information per Serving:

Calories: 109
Fat: 6.6g
Carbohydrates: 12g
Fiber: 3.5g
Sugar: 7.8g
Protein: 2.9g
Sodium: 23mg

Blueberries & Spinach Salad

Servings: 4
Preparation Time: 15 minutes

Ingredients:

For Salad:

- 6 cups fresh baby spinach
- 1 ½ cups fresh blueberries
- ¼ cup onion, sliced
- ¼ cup almond, sliced
- ¼ cup feta cheese, crumbled

For Dressing:

- 1/3 cup olive oil
- 2 tablespoons fresh lemon juice
- ¼ teaspoon liquid stevia
- 1/8 teaspoon garlic powder
- Salt, as required

Instructions:

1. **For Salad**: in a bowl, add the spinach, berries, onion and almonds and mix.
2. **For Dressing**: in another small bowl, add all the ingredients and beat until well blended.
3. Place the dressing over salad and gently toss to coat well.
4. Serve immediately.

Nutritional Information per Serving:

Calories: 250
Fat: 22.2g
Carbohydrates: 12g
Fiber: 3.2g
Sugar: 6.7g
Protein: 4.5g
Sodium: 181mg

Mixed Berries Salad

Servings: 4
Preparation Time: 15 minutes

Ingredients:

- 1 cup fresh strawberries, hulled and sliced
- ½ cups fresh blackberries
- ½ cup fresh blueberries
- ½ cup fresh raspberries
- 6 cup fresh arugula
- 2 tablespoons extra-virgin olive oil
- Salt and ground black pepper, as required

Instructions:

1. In a salad bowl, place all the ingredients and toss to coat well.
2. Serve immediately.

Nutritional Information per Serving:

Calories: 105
Fat: 20.2g
Carbohydrates: 12g
Fiber: 3.2g
Sugar: 6.7g
Protein: 4.5g
Sodium: mg

Kale & Citrus Fruit Salad

Servings: 2
Preparation Time: 15 minutes

Ingredients:

For Salad:

- 3 cups fresh kale, tough ribs removed and torn
- 1 orange, peeled and segmented
- 1 grapefruit, peeled and segmented
- 2 tablespoons unsweetened dried cranberries
- ¼ teaspoon white sesame seeds

For Dressing:

- 2 tablespoons extra-virgin olive oil
- 2 tablespoons fresh orange juice
- 1 teaspoon Dijon mustard
- ½ teaspoon raw honey
- Salt and ground black pepper, as required

Instructions:

1. **For Salad**: in a salad bowl, place all ingredients and mix.
2. **For Dressing**: place all ingredients in another bowl and beat until well combined.
3. Place dressing on top of salad and toss to coat well.
4. Serve immediately.

Nutritional Information per Serving:

Calories: 256
Fat: 14.5g
Carbohydrates: 25g
Fiber: 4.8g
Sugar: 16g
Protein: 4.6g
Sodium: 150mg

Kale, Apple & Cranberry Salad

Servings: 4
Preparation Time: 15 minutes

Ingredients:

- 6 cups fresh baby kale
- 3 large apples, cored and sliced
- ¼ cup unsweetened dried cranberries
- ¼ cup almonds, sliced
- 2 tablespoons extra-virgin olive oil
- 1 tablespoon raw honey
- Salt and ground black pepper, as required

Instructions:

1. In a salad bowl, place all the ingredients and toss to coat well.
2. Serve immediately.

Nutritional Information per Serving:

Calories: 153
Fat: 10.3g
Carbohydrates: 40g
Fiber: 6.6g
Sugar: 20g
Protein: 4.7g
Sodium: 109mg

Rocket, Beat & Orange Salad

Servings: 4
Preparation Time: 15 minutes

Ingredients:

- 3 large oranges, peeled, seeded and sectioned
- 2 beets, trimmed, peeled and sliced
- 6 cups fresh rocket
- ¼ cup walnuts, chopped
- 3 tablespoons olive oil
- Pinch of salt

Instructions:

1. In a salad bowl, place all ingredients and gently toss to coat.
2. Serve immediately.

Nutritional Information per Serving:

Calories: 233
Fat: 15.6g
Carbohydrates: 23.1g
Fiber: 5.3g
Sugar: 17.6g
Protein: 4.8g
Sodium: 86mg

Cucumber & Tomato Salad

Servings: 6
Preparation Time: 15 minutes

Ingredients:

For Salad:

- 3 large English cucumbers, sliced thinly
- 2 cups tomatoes, chopped
- 6 cup lettuce, torn

For Dressing:

- 4 tablespoons olive oil
- 2 tablespoons balsamic vinegar
- 1 tablespoon fresh lemon juice
- Salt and ground black pepper, as required

Instructions:

1. **For Salad**: in a large bowl, add the cucumbers, onion and dill and mix.
2. **For Dressing**: in a small bowl, add all the ingredients and beat until well combined.
3. Place the dressing over the salad and toss to coat well.
4. Serve immediately.

Nutritional Information per Serving:

Calories: 86
Fat: 7.3g
Carbohydrates: 5.1g
Fiber: 9.8g
Sugar: 2.8g
Protein: 1.1g
Sodium: 27mg

Mixed Veggie Salad

Servings: 6
Preparation Time: 20 minutes

Ingredients:

For Dressing:

- I small avocado, peeled, pitted and chopped
- ¼ cup low-fat plain Greek yogurt
- I small yellow onion, chopped
- I garlic clove, chopped
- 2 tablespoons fresh parsley
- 2 tablespoons fresh lemon juice

For Salad:

- 6 cups fresh spinach, shredded
- 2 medium zucchini, cut into thin slices
- ½ cup celery, sliced
- ½ cup red bell pepper, seeded and sliced thinly
- ½ cup yellow onion, sliced thinly
- ½ cup cucumber, sliced thinly
- ½ cup cherry tomatoes, halved
- ¼ cup Kalamata olives, pitted
- ½ cup feta cheese, crumbled

Instructions:

1. **For Dressing**: in a food processor, add all the ingredients and pulse until smooth.
2. **For Salad**: in a salad bowl, add all the ingredients and mix well.
3. Pour the dressing over salad and gently, toss to coat well.
4. Serve immediately.

Nutritional Information per Serving:

Calories: 152
Fat: 10.3g
Carbohydrates: 12g
Fiber: 4.8g
Sugar: 4.8g
Protein: 5.4g
Sodium: 238mg

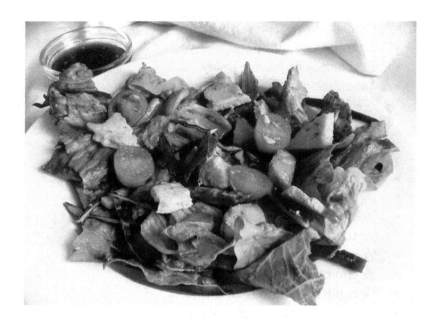

Eggs & Veggie Salad

Servings: 8
Preparation Time: 15 minutes

Ingredients:

For Salad:

- 2 large English cucumbers, sliced thinly sliced
- 2 cups tomatoes, chopped
- 8 hard-boiled eggs, peeled and sliced
- 8 cups fresh baby spinach

For Dressing:

- 4 tablespoons olive oil
- 2 tablespoons balsamic vinegar
- 1 tablespoon fresh lemon juice
- Salt and ground black pepper, as required

Instructions:

1. **For Salad**: in a salad bowl, add the cucumbers, onion and dill and mix.
2. **For Dressing**: in a small bowl, add all the ingredients and beat until well blended.
3. Place the dressing over the salad and toss to coat well.
4. Serve immediately.

Nutritional Information per Serving:

Calories: 150
Fat: 11.7g
Carbohydrates: 6g
Fiber: 1.6g
Sugar: 3g
Protein: 7.3g
Sodium: 109mg

Tofu & Veggie Salad

Servings: 8
Preparation Time: 20 minutes

Ingredients:

For Dressing:

- ¼ cup balsamic vinegar
- ¼ cup low-sodium soy sauce
- 2 tablespoons water
- 1 teaspoon sesame oil, toasted
- 1 teaspoon Sriracha
- 3-4 drops liquid stevia

For Salad:

- 1 ½ pounds baked firm tofu, cubed
- 2 large zucchinis, sliced thinly
- 2 large yellow bell peppers, seeded and sliced thinly
- 3 cups cherry tomatoes, halved
- 2 cups radishes, sliced thinly
- 2 cups purple cabbage, shredded
- 10 cups fresh baby spinach

Instructions:

1. **For Dressing**: in a bowl, add all the ingredients and beat until well combined.
2. Divide the chickpeas, tofu and vegetables into serving bowls.
3. Drizzle with dressing and serve immediately.

Nutritional Information per Serving:

Calories: 122
Fat: 4.7g
Carbohydrates: 13.1g
Fiber: 4.6g
Sugar: 7g
Protein: 10.8g
Sodium: 511mg

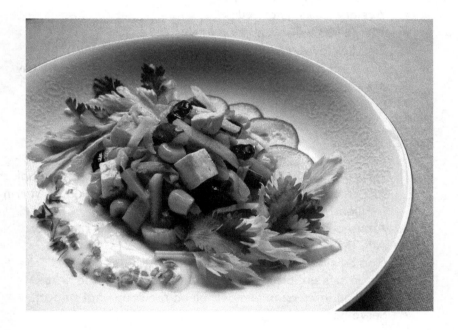

Kale & Carrot Soup

Servings: 5
Preparation Time: 15 minutes
Cooking Time: 40 minutes

Ingredients:

- 2 tablespoons extra-virgin olive oil
- 4 medium carrots, chopped
- 2 celery stalks, chopped
- 1 large red onion, chopped finely
- 2 garlic cloves, crushed
- ½ pound curly kale, tough ribs removed and chopped finely
- 4½ cups homemade low-sodium vegetable broth
- Salt and ground black pepper, as required

Instructions:

1. Heat the oil in a large soup pan over medium heat and cook the carrot, celery, onion and garlic for about 8-10 minutes, stirring frequently.
2. Add the kale and cook for about 5 minutes, stirring twice.
3. Add the broth and bring to a boil.
4. Cook, partially covered for about 20 minutes.
5. Stir in salt and black pepper and remove from the heat.
6. With an immersion blender, blend the soup until smooth.
7. Serve hot.

Nutritional Information per Serving:

Calories: 140
Fat: 6.9g
Carbohydrates: 13g
Fiber: 2.7g
Sugar: 4.4g
Protein: 6.6g
Sodium: 778mg

Cheesy Mushroom Soup

Servings: 4
Preparation Time: 15 minutes
Cooking Time: 15 minutes

Ingredients:

- 2 tablespoons olive oil
- 4 ounces fresh baby Portobello mushroom, sliced
- 4 ounces fresh white button mushrooms, sliced
- ½ cup yellow onion, chopped
- ½ teaspoon salt
- 1 teaspoon garlic, chopped
- 3 cups low-sodium vegetable broth
- 1 cup low-fat cheddar cheese

Instructions:

1. In a medium pan, heat the oil over medium heat and cook the mushrooms and onion with salt for about 5-7 minutes, stirring frequently.
2. Add the garlic, and sauté for about 1-2 minutes.
3. Stir in the broth and remove from the heat.
4. With a stick blender, blend the soup until mushrooms are chopped very finely.
5. In the pan, add the cheddar cheese and stir to combine.
6. Place the pan over medium heat and cook for about 3-5 minutes.
7. Remove from the heat and serve immediately.

Nutritional Information per Serving:

Calories: 204
Fat: 16.5g
Carbohydrates: 4.6g
Fiber: 0.9g
Sugar: 1.7g
Protein: 10.5g
Sodium: 523mg

Spinach & Mushroom Stew

Servings: 4
Preparation Time: 15 minutes
Cooking Time: 30 minutes

Ingredients:

- 2 tablespoons olive oil
- 2 onions, chopped
- 3 garlic cloves, minced
- ½ pound fresh button mushrooms, chopped
- ¼ pound fresh shiitake mushrooms, chopped
- ¼ pound fresh spinach, chopped
- Sea salt and freshly ground black pepper, as required
- ¼ cup low-sodium vegetable broth
- ½ cup coconut milk
- 2 tablespoons fresh parsley, chopped

Instructions:

1. In a large wok, heat oil over medium heat and sauté the onion and garlic for 4-5 minutes.
2. Add the mushrooms, salt, and black pepper and cook for 4-5 minutes.
3. Add the spinach, broth and coconut milk and bring to a gentle boil.
4. Simmer for 4-5 minutes or until desired doneness.
5. Stir in the parsley and remove from heat.
6. Serve hot.

Nutritional Information per Serving:

Calories: 181
Fat: 14.6g
Carbohydrates: 11.5g
Fiber: 3.4g
Sugar: 5g
Protein: 5.1g
Sodium: 90mg

Veggie Stew

Servings: 4
Preparation Time: 20 minutes
Cooking Time: 35 minutes

Ingredients:

- 2 tablespoons olive oil
- 1 yellow onion, chopped
- 2 teaspoons fresh ginger, grated
- 1 teaspoon ground turmeric
- 1 teaspoon ground cumin
- Salt and ground black pepper, as required
- 1-2 cups water, divided
- 1 cup cabbage, shredded
- 1 cup broccoli, chopped
- 2 large carrots, peeled and sliced

Instructions:

1. In a large soup pan, heat the oil over medium heat and sauté onion for about 5 minutes.
2. Stir in the ginger and spices and sauté for about 1 minute.
3. Add 1 cup of water and bring to a boil.
4. Reduce the heat to medium-low and cook for about 10 minutes.
5. Add the vegetables and enough water that covers the half of vegetable mixture and stir to combine.
6. Increase the heat to medium-high and bring to a boil.
7. Reduce the heat to medium-low and cook, covered for about 10-15 minutes, stirring occasionally.
8. Serve hot.

Nutritional Information per Serving:

Calories: 105
Fat: 7.4g
Carbohydrates: 9g
Fiber: 2.8g
Sugar: 4g
Protein: 1.7g
Sodium: 77mg

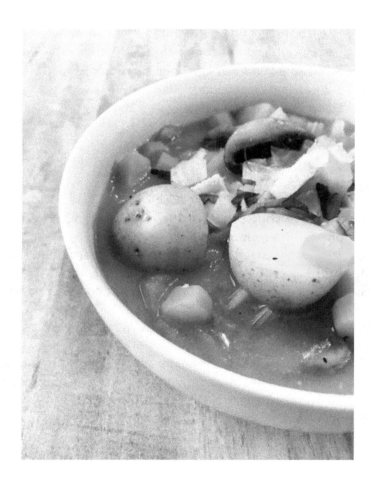

Tofu & Mushroom Soup

Servings: 3
Preparation Time: 15 minutes
Cooking Time: 25 minutes

Ingredients:

- 3 tablespoons vegetable oil, divided
- 1 shallot, minced
- 1 ounce fresh ginger, minced
- 2 garlic cloves, minced
- 5½ ounces coconut milk
- 1 Roma tomato, chopped
- 1 lemongrass stalk, halved crosswise
- 6 ounces fresh mushrooms, sliced
- 14 ounces extra-firm tofu, pressed, drained and cut into ½-inch cubes
- Ground black pepper, as required
- 1 scallion, sliced
- 1 tablespoon fresh cilantro, chopped

Instructions:

1. In a pan, heat 2 tablespoons of oil over medium-high heat and sauté the shallot, ginger, garlic and a pinch of salt for about 1-2 minutes.
2. Add coconut milk and remaining water and bring to a boil.
3. Add the tomato and lemongrass and stir to combine.
4. Adjust the heat to low and simmer for about 8-10 minutes.
5. Meanwhile, in a large non-stick wok, heat the remaining oil over medium-high heat and cook the mushrooms, tofu, pinch of salt and black pepper for about 5-8 minutes, stirring occasionally.
6. Remove the lemongrass stalk from pan of soup and discard it.
7. Divide the cooked mushrooms and tofu into serving bowls evenly.
8. Top with hot soup and serve with the garnishing of scallion and cilantro.

Nutritional Information per Serving:

Calories: 344
Fat: 28.7g
Carbohydrates: 8.7g
Fiber: 1.5g
Sugar: 3.6g
Protein: 16.1g
Sodium: 33mg

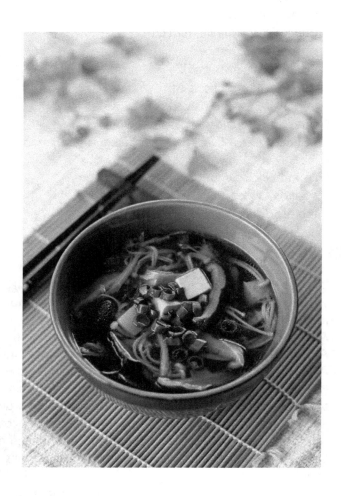

Tofu & Bell Pepper Stew

Servings: 6
Preparation Time: 15 minutes
Cooking Time: 15 minutes

Ingredients:

- 2 tablespoons garlic
- 1 jalapeño pepper, seeded and chopped
- 1 (16-ounce) jar roasted red peppers, rinsed, drained and chopped
- 2 cups homemade low-sodium vegetable broth
- 2 cups filtered water
- 1 medium green bell pepper, seeded and sliced thinly
- 1 medium red bell pepper, seeded and sliced thinly
- 1 (16-ounce) package extra-firm tofu, drained and cubed
- 1 (10-ounce) package frozen baby spinach, thawed

Instructions:

1. Add the garlic, jalapeño pepper and roasted red peppers in a food processor and pulse until smooth.
2. In a large pan, add the puree, broth and water over medium-high heat and cook until boiling.
3. Add the bell peppers and tofu and stir to combine.
4. Reduce the heat to medium and cook for about 5 minutes.
5. Stir in the spinach and cook for about 5 minutes.
6. Serve hot.

Nutritional Information per Serving:

Calories: 132
Fat: 5g
Carbohydrates: 14g
Fiber: 3.1g
Sugar: 6.7g
Protein: 11.5g
Sodium: 75mg

Carrot Soup with Tempeh

Servings: 6
Preparation Time: 15 minutes
Cooking Time: 45 minutes

Ingredients:

- ¼ cup olive oil, divided
- 1 large yellow onion, chopped
- Salt, as required
- 2 pounds carrots, peeled and cut into ½-inch rounds
- 2 tablespoons fresh dill, chopped
- 4½ cups low-sodium vegetable broth
- 12 ounces tempeh, cut into ½-inch cubes
- ¼ cup tomato paste
- 1 teaspoon fresh lemon juice

Instructions:

1. In a large soup pan, heat 2 tablespoons of the oil over medium heat and cook the onion with salt for about 6-8 minutes, stirring frequently.
2. Add the carrots and stir to combine.
3. Lower the heat to low and cook, covered for about 5 minutes, stirring frequently.
4. Add in the broth and bring to a boil over high heat.
5. Lower the heat to a low and simmer, covered for about 30 minutes.
6. Meanwhile, in a wok, heat the remaining oil over medium-high heat and cook the tempeh for about 3-5 minutes.
7. Stir in the dill and cook for about 1 minute.
8. Remove from the heat.
9. Remove the pan of soup from heat and stir in tomato paste and lemon juice.
10. With an immersion blender, blend the soup until smooth and creamy.
11. Serve the soup hot with the topping of tempeh.

Nutritional Information per Serving:

Calories: 294
Fat: 15.7g
Carbohydrates: 20g
Fiber: 4.9g
Sugar: 10g
Protein: 16.4g
Sodium: 273mg

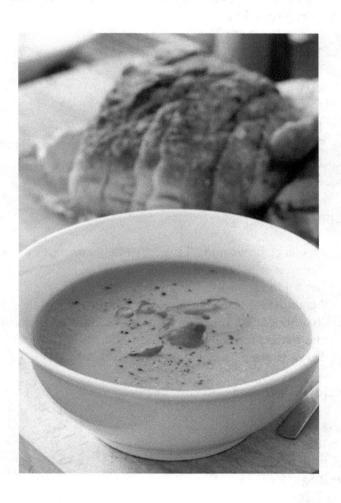

Vegetarian Burgers

Servings: 4
Preparation Time: 15 minutes
Cooking Time: 16 minutes

Ingredients:

- 1-pound firm tofu, drained, pressed, and crumbled
- ¾ cup rolled oats
- ¼ cup flaxseeds
- 2 cups frozen spinach, thawed
- 1 medium onion, chopped finely
- 4 garlic cloves, minced
- 1 teaspoon ground cumin
- 1 teaspoon red pepper flakes, crushed
- Sea salt and freshly ground black pepper, as required
- 2 tablespoons olive oil
- 6 cups fresh salad greens

Instructions:

1. In a large bowl, add all the ingredients except oil and salad greens and mix until well combined.
2. Set aside for about 10 minutes.
3. Make desired size patties from mixture.
4. In a nonstick frying pan, heat the oil over medium heat and cook the patties for 6-8 minutes per side.
5. Serve these patties alongside the salad greens.

Nutritional Information per Serving:

Calories: 214
Fat: 11.8g
Carbohydrates: 4.6g
Fiber: 2.5g
Sugar: 2.2g
Protein: 24.6g
Sodium: 80mg

Cauliflower with Peas

Servings: 4
Preparation Time: 15 minutes
Cooking Time: 15 minutes

Ingredients:

- 2 medium tomatoes, chopped
- ¼ cup water
- 2 tablespoons olive oil
- 3 garlic cloves, minced
- ½ tablespoon fresh ginger, minced
- 1 teaspoon ground cumin
- 2 teaspoons ground coriander
- 1 teaspoon cayenne pepper
- ¼ teaspoon ground turmeric
- 2 cups cauliflower, chopped
- 1 cup fresh green peas, shelled
- Salt and ground black pepper, as required
- ½ cup warm water

Instructions:

1. In a blender, add tomato and ¼ cup of water and pulse until smooth puree forms. Set aside.
2. In a large wok, heat the oil over medium heat and sauté the garlic, ginger, green chilies and spices for about 1 minute.
3. Add the cauliflower, peas and tomato puree and cook, stirring for about 3-4 minutes.
4. Add the warm water and bring to a boil.
5. Reduce the heat to medium-low and cook, covered for about 8-10 minutes or until vegetables are done completely.
6. Serve hot.

Nutritional Information per Serving:

Calories: 163
Fat: 10.1g
Carbohydrates: 16.1g
Fiber: 5.6g
Sugar: 6g
Protein: 6g
Sodium: 79mg

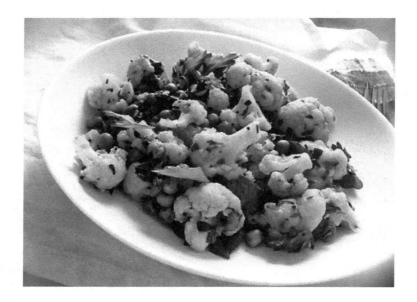

Broccoli with Bell Peppers

Servings: 6
Preparation Time: 15 minutes
Cooking Time: 10 minutes

Ingredients:

- 2 tablespoons olive oil
- 4 garlic cloves, minced
- 1 large white onion, sliced
- 2 cups small broccoli florets
- 3 red bell peppers, seeded and sliced
- ¼ cup low-sodium vegetable broth
- Salt and ground black pepper, as required

Instructions:

1. In a large wok, heat the oil over medium heat and sauté the garlic for about 1 minute.
2. Add the onion, broccoli and bell peppers and stir fry for about 5 minutes.
3. Add the broth and stir fry for about 4 minutes more.
4. Serve hot.

Nutritional Information per Serving:

Calories: 84
Fat: 5g
Carbohydrates: 9.6g
Fiber: 2.2g
Sugar: 4.6g
Protein: 2.1g
Sodium: 72mg

3-Veggies Medley

Servings: 6
Preparation Time: 25 minutes
Cooking Time: 15 minutes

Ingredients:

- 1 tablespoon olive oil
- 1 small yellow onion, chopped
- 1 teaspoon fresh thyme, chopped
- 1 garlic clove, minced
- 8 ounces fresh mushrooms, sliced
- 1-pound Brussels sprouts
- 3 cups fresh spinach
- Salt and ground black pepper, as required

Instructions:

1. In a large wok, heat the oil over medium heat and sauté the onion for about 3-4 minutes.
2. Add the thyme and garlic and sauté for about 1 minute.
3. Add the mushrooms and cook for about 15 minutes or until caramelized.
4. Add the Brussels sprouts and cook for about 2-3 minutes.
5. Stir in the spinach and cook for about 3-4 minutes.
6. Stir in the salt and black pepper and remove from the heat.
7. Serve hot.

Nutritional Information per Serving:

Calories: 70
Fat: 2.8g
Carbohydrates: 10g
Fiber: 3.9g
Sugar: 2.8g
Protein: 4.4g
Sodium: 61mg

3 Veggies Combo

Servings: 4
Preparation Time: 15 minutes
Cooking Time: 10 minutes

Ingredients:

- 1 tablespoon olive oil
- ½ cup onion, sliced
- ½ cup red bell pepper, seeded and julienned
- ½ cup orange bell pepper, seeded and julienned
- 1½ cups yellow squash, sliced
- 1½ cups zucchini, sliced
- 1½ teaspoons garlic, minced
- ¼ cup water
- Salt and ground black pepper, as required

Instructions:

1. In a large wok, heat the oil over medium-high heat and sauté the onion, bell peppers and squash for about 4-5 minutes.
2. Add the garlic and sauté for about 1 minute.
3. Add the remaining ingredients and stir to combine.
4. Reduce the heat to medium and cook for about 3-4 minutes, stirring occasionally.
5. Serve hot.

Nutritional Information per Serving:

Calories: 65
Fat: 3.8g
Carbohydrates: 7.7g
Fiber: 1.7g
Sugar: 3.6g
Protein: 1.7g
Sodium: 50mg

Bok Choy & Mushroom Stir Fry

Servings: 4
Preparation Time: 15 minutes
Cooking Time: 10 minutes

Ingredients:

- 1 pound baby bok choy
- 4 teaspoons olive oil
- 1 teaspoon fresh ginger, minced
- 2 garlic cloves, chopped
- 5 ounces fresh mushrooms, sliced
- 2 tablespoons red wine
- 2 tablespoons soy sauce
- Ground black pepper, as required

Instructions:

1. Trim bases of bok choy and separate outer leaves from stalks, leaving the smallest inner leaves attached.
2. In a large cast-iron wok, heat the oil over medium-high heat and sauté the ginger and garlic for about 1 minute.
3. Stir in the mushrooms and cook for about 4-5 minutes, stirring frequently.
4. Stir in the bok choy leaves and stalks and cook for about 1 minute, tossing with tongs.
5. Stir in the wine, soy sauce and black pepper and cook for about 2-3 minutes, tossing occasionally.
6. Serve hot.

Nutritional Information per Serving:

Calories: 77
Fat: 5g
Carbohydrates: 5.3g
Fiber: 1.6g
Sugar: 2.2g
Protein: 3.5g
Sodium: 527mg

Broccoli with Bell Peppers

Servings: 6
Preparation Time: 10 minutes
Cooking Time: 10 minutes

Ingredients:

- 2 tablespoons olive oil
- 4 garlic cloves, minced
- 1 large white onion, sliced
- 2 cups small broccoli florets
- 3 red bell peppers, seeded and sliced
- ¼ cup low-sodium vegetable broth
- Salt and ground black pepper, as required

Instructions:

1. In a large wok, heat oil over medium heat and sauté the garlic for about 1 minute.
2. Add the onion, broccoli and bell peppers and cook for about 5 minutes, stirring frequently.
3. Stir in the broth and cook for about 4 minutes, stirring frequently.
4. Stir in the salt and black pepper and remove from the heat.
5. Serve hot.

Nutritional Information per Serving:

Calories: 170
Fat: 3g
Carbohydrates: 6g
Fiber: 2g
Sugar: 1g
Protein: 2g
Sodium: 347mg

Stuffed Zucchini

Servings: 8
Preparation Time: 15 minutes
Cooking Time: 18 minutes

Ingredients:

- 4 medium zucchinis, halved lengthwise
- 1 cup red bell pepper, seeded and minced
- ½ cup Kalamata olives, pitted and minced
- ½ cup tomatoes, minced
- 1 teaspoon garlic, minced
- 1 tablespoon dried oregano, crushed
- Salt and ground black pepper, as required
- ½ cup feta cheese, crumbled
- ¼ cup fresh parsley, chopped finely

Instructions:

1. Preheat your oven to 350 degrees F.
2. Grease a large baking sheet.
3. With a melon baller, scoop out the flesh of each zucchini half. Discard the flesh.
4. In a bowl, mix together bell pepper, olives, tomato, garlic, oregano and black pepper.
5. Stuff each zucchini half with veggie mixture evenly.
6. Arrange zucchini halves onto the prepared baking sheet and bake for approximately 15 minutes.
7. Now, set the oven to broiler on high.
8. Top each zucchini half with feta cheese and broil for about 3 minutes.
9. Garnish with parsley and serve hot.

Nutritional Information per Serving:

Calories: 60
Fat: 3.2g
Carbohydrates: 6.4g
Fiber: 2g
Sugar: 3.2g
Protein: 3g
Sodium: 209mg

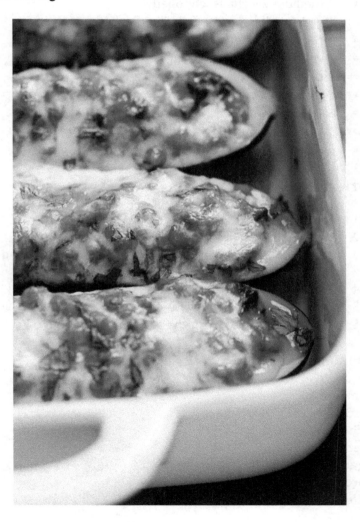

Zucchini & Bell Pepper Curry

Servings: 6
Preparation Time: 20 minutes
Cooking Time: 20 minutes

Ingredients:

- 2 medium zucchinis, chopped
- 1 green bell pepper, seeded and cubed
- 1 red bell pepper, seeded and cubed
- 1 yellow onion, sliced thinly
- 2 tablespoons olive oil
- 2 teaspoons curry powder
- Salt and ground black pepper, as required
- ¼ cup homemade low-sodium vegetable broth
- ¼ cup fresh cilantro, chopped

Instructions:

1. Preheat your oven to 375 degrees F.
2. Lightly grease a large baking dish.
3. In a large bowl, add all ingredients except cilantro and mix until well combined.
4. Transfer the vegetable mixture into the prepared baking dish.
5. Bake for approximately 15-20 minutes.
6. Serve immediately with the garnishing of cilantro.

Nutritional Information per Serving:

Calories: 60
Fat: 3.2g
Carbohydrates: 6.4g
Fiber: 2g
Sugar: 3.2g
Protein: 3g
Sodium: 209mg

Zucchini Noodles with Mushroom Sauce

Servings: 5
Preparation Time: 20 minutes
Cooking Time: 15 minutes

Ingredients:

For Mushroom Sauce:

- 1 ½ tablespoons olive oil
- 1 large garlic clove, minced
- 1 ¼ cups fresh button mushrooms, sliced
- ¼ cup homemade low-sodium vegetable broth
- ¼ cup cream
- Salt and ground black pepper, as required

For Zucchini Noodles:

- 3 large zucchinis, spiralized with blade C
- ¼ cup fresh parsley leaves, chopped

Instructions:

1. For mushroom sauce: In a large wok, heat the oil over medium heat and sauté the garlic for about 1 minute.
2. Stir in the mushrooms and cook for about 6-8 minutes.
3. Stir in the broth and cook for about 2 minutes, stirring continuously.
4. Stir in the cream, salt and black pepper and cook for about 1 minute.
5. Meanwhile, for the zucchini noodles: in a large pan of boiling water, add the zucchini noodles and cook for about 2-3 minutes.
6. With a slotted spoon, transfer the zucchini noodles into a colander and immediately rinse under cold running water.
7. Drain the zucchini noodles well and transfer onto a large paper towel-lined plate to drain.
8. Divide the zucchini noodles onto serving plates evenly.

9. Remove the mushroom sauce from the heat and place over zucchini noodles evenly.
10. Serve immediately with the garnishing of parsley.

Nutritional Information per Serving:

Calories: 77
Fat: 4.6g
Carbohydrates: 7.9g
Fiber: 2.4g
Sugar: 4g
Protein: 3.4g
Sodium: 120mg

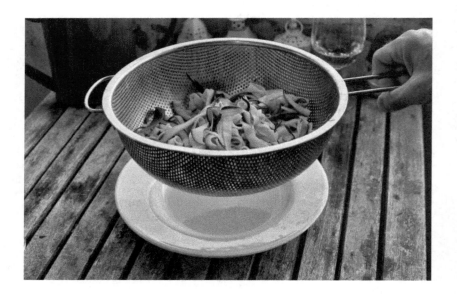

Squash Casserole

Servings: 8
Preparation Time: 15 minutes
Cooking Time: 55 minutes

Ingredients:

- ¼ cup plus 2 tablespoons olive oil, divided
- 1 small yellow onion, chopped
- 3 summer squashes, sliced
- 4 eggs, beaten
- 3 cups low-fat cheddar cheese, shredded and divided
- 2 tablespoons unsweetened almond milk
- 2-3 tablespoons almond flour
- 2 tablespoons Erythritol
- Salt and ground black pepper, as required

Instructions:

1. Preheat your oven to 375 degrees F.
2. In a large wok, heat 2 tablespoons of oil over medium heat and cook the onion and squash for about 8-10 minutes, stirring occasionally.
3. Remove the wok from the heat.
4. Place the eggs, 1 cup of cheddar cheese, almond milk, almond flour, Erythritol, salt and black pepper in a large bowl and mix until well combined.
5. Add the squash mixture, and remaining oil and stir to combine.
6. Transfer the mixture into a large casserole dish and sprinkle with the remaining cheddar cheese.
7. Bake for approximately 35-45 minutes.
8. Remove the casserole dish from oven and set aside for about 5-10 minutes before serving.
9. Cut into 8 equal-sized portions and serve.

Nutritional Information per Serving:

Calories: 284
Fat: 22.8g
Carbohydrates: 5g
Fiber: 1.2g
Sugar: 1.9g
Protein: 15.8g
Sodium: 361mg

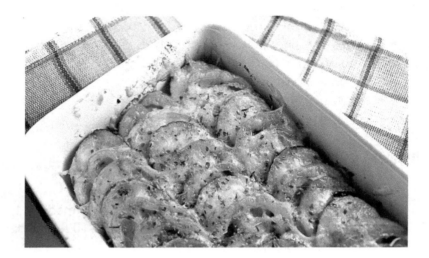

Veggies & Walnut Loaf

Servings: 10
Preparation Time: 15 minutes
Cooking Time: 1 hour 10 minutes

Ingredients:

- 1 tablespoon olive oil
- 2 yellow onions, chopped
- 2 garlic cloves, minced
- 1 teaspoon dried rosemary, crushed
- 1 cup walnuts, chopped
- 2 large carrots, peeled and chopped
- 1 large celery stalk, chopped
- 1 large green bell pepper, seeded and chopped
- 1 cup fresh button mushrooms, chopped
- 5 large eggs
- 1 ¼ cups almond flour
- Salt and ground black pepper, as required

Instructions:

1. Preheat your oven to 350-degree F.
2. Line 2 loaf pans with lightly greased parchment papers.
3. In a large wok, heat the olive oil over medium heat and sauté the onion for about 4-5 minutes.
4. Add the garlic and rosemary and sauté for about 1 minute.
5. Add the walnuts and vegetables and cook for about 3–4 minutes.
6. Remove the wok from heat and transfer the mixture into a large bowl.
7. Set aside to cool slightly.
8. In another mixing bowl, add the eggs, flour, sea salt, and black pepper, and beat until well combined.
9. Add the egg mixture into the bowl with vegetable mixture and mix until well combined.
10. Divide the mixture into prepared loaf pans evenly.
11. Bake for approximately 50–60 minutes or until top becomes golden brown.

12. Remove from the oven and set aside to cool slightly.
13. Carefully invert the loaves onto a platter.
14. Cut into desired sized slices and serve.

Nutritional Information per Serving:

Calories: 195
Fat: 15.5g
Carbohydrates: 9.1g
Fiber: 3.5g
Sugar: 2.5g
Protein: 6.8g
Sodium: 32mg

Tofu & Veggie Burgers

Servings: 2
Preparation Time: 20 minutes
Cooking Time: 8 minutes

Ingredients:

For Patties:

- ½ cup firm tofu, pressed and drained
- 1 medium carrot, peeled and gated
- 1 tablespoon onion, chopped
- 1 tablespoon scallion, chopped
- 1 tablespoon fresh parsley, chopped
- ½ garlic clove, minced
- 2 teaspoons low-sodium soy sauce
- 1 tablespoon arrowroot flour
- 1 teaspoon nutritional yeast flakes
- ½ teaspoon Dijon mustard
- 1 teaspoon paprika
- ¼ teaspoon ground turmeric
- ½ teaspoon ground black pepper
- 2 tablespoons olive oil

For Serving:

- ½ cup cherry tomatoes, halved
- 2 cup fresh baby greens

Instructions:

1. For patties: in a bowl, add the tofu and with a fork, mash well.
2. Add the remaining ingredients except for oil and mix until well combined.
3. Make 4 equal-sized patties from the mixture.
4. Heat the oil in a frying pan over low heat and cook the patties for about 4 minutes per side.

5. Divide the avocado, tomatoes and greens onto serving plates.
6. Top each plate with 2 patties and serve.

Nutritional Information per Serving:

Calories: 198
Fat: 17g
Carbohydrates: 7.9g
Fiber: 2.7g
Sugar: 2.7g
Protein: 7.2g
Sodium: 341mg

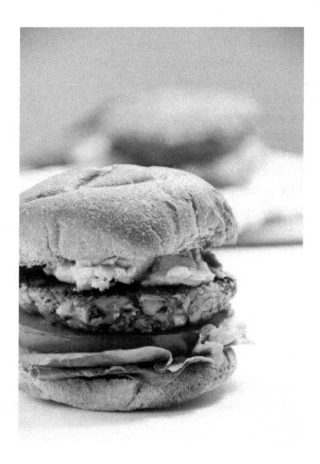

Tofu & Veggie Lettuce Wraps

Servings: 4
Preparation Time: 15 minutes
Cooking Time: 6 minutes

Ingredients:

For Wraps:

- 1 tablespoon olive oil
- 14 ounces extra-firm tofu, drained, pressed and cut into cubes
- 1 teaspoon curry powder
- Salt, as required
- 8 lettuce leaves
- 1 small carrot, peeled and julienned
- ½ cup radishes, sliced
- 2 tablespoons fresh cilantro, chopped

For Sauce:

- ½ cup creamy peanut butter
- 1 tablespoon maple syrup
- 2 tablespoons low-sodium soy sauce
- 2 tablespoons fresh lime juice
- ¼ teaspoon red pepper flakes, crushed
- ¼ cup water

Instructions:

1. For tofu: in a wok, heat the oil over medium heat and cook the tofu, curry powder and a little salt for about 5-6 minutes or until golden brown, stirring frequently.
2. Remove from the heat and set aside to cool slightly.
3. Meanwhile, for sauce: in a bowl, add all the ingredients and beat until smooth.
4. Arrange the lettuce leaves onto serving plates.
5. Divide the tofu, carrot, radish and peanuts over each leaf evenly.

6. Garnish with cilantro and serve alongside the peanut sauce.

Nutritional Information per Serving:

Calories: 381
Fat: 28.5g
Carbohydrates: 18g
Fiber: 4.4g
Sugar: 9g
Protein: 19.4g
Sodium: 657mg

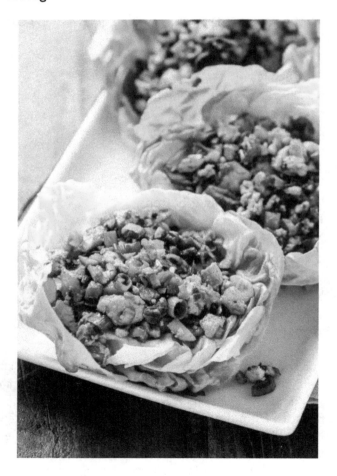

Tofu with Kale

Servings: 2
Preparation Time: 15 minutes
Cooking Time: 10 minutes

Ingredients:

- 1 tablespoon extra-virgin olive oil
- ½ pound tofu, pressed, drained and cubed
- 1 teaspoon fresh ginger, minced
- 1 garlic clove, minced
- ¼ teaspoon red pepper flakes, crushed
- 6 ounces fresh kale, tough ribs removed and chopped finely
- 1 tablespoon low-sodium soy sauce

Instructions:

1. In a large non-stick wok, heat olive oil over medium-high heat and stir-fry the tofu for about 3-3 minutes.
2. Add the ginger, garlic and red pepper flakes and cook for about 1 minute, stirring continuously.
3. Stir in the kale and soy sauce and stir-fry for about 4-5 minutes.
4. Serve hot.

Nutritional Information per Serving:

Calories: 190
Fat: 11.8g
Carbohydrates: 11g
Fiber: 3g
Sugar: 1.3g
Protein: 12.8g
Sodium: 487mg

Tofu with Broccoli

Servings: 4
Preparation Time: 20 minutes
Cooking Time: 25 minutes

Ingredients:

For Tofu:

- 14 ounces firm tofu, drained, pressed and cut into 1-inch slices
- 1/3 cup arrowroot starch, divided
- ¼ cup olive oil
- 1 teaspoon fresh ginger, grated
- 1 medium onion, sliced thinly
- 3 tablespoons low-sodium soy sauce
- 2 tablespoons balsamic vinegar
- 1 tablespoon maple syrup
- ½ cup water

For Steamed Broccoli:

- 2 cups broccoli florets

Instructions:

1. In a shallow bowl, place ¼ cup of the arrowroot starch.
2. Add the tofu cubes and coat with arrowroot starch.
3. In a cast-iron wok, heat the olive oil over medium heat and cook the tofu cubes for about 8-10 minutes or until golden from all sides.
4. With a slotted spoon, transfer the tofu cubes onto a plate. Set aside.
5. In the same wok, add ginger and sauté for about 1 minute.
6. Add the onions and sauté for about 2-3 minutes.
7. Add the soy sauce, vinegar and maple syrup and bring to a gentle simmer.
8. In the meantime, in a small bowl, dissolve the remaining arrowroot starch in water.

9. Slowly, add the arrowroot starch mixture into the sauce, stirring continuously.
10. Stir in the cooked tofu and cook for about 1 minute.
11. Meanwhile, in a large pan of water, arrange a steamer basket and bring to a boil.
12. Adjust the heat to medium-low.
13. Place the broccoli florets in the steamer basket and steam, covered for about 5-6 minutes.
14. Remove from the heat and drain the broccoli completely.
15. Transfer the broccoli into the wok of tofu and stir to combine.
16. Serve hot.

Nutritional Information per Serving:

Calories: 230
Fat: 17g
Carbohydrates: 11g
Fiber: 2.9g
Sugar: 6g
Protein: 10.9g
Sodium: 692mg

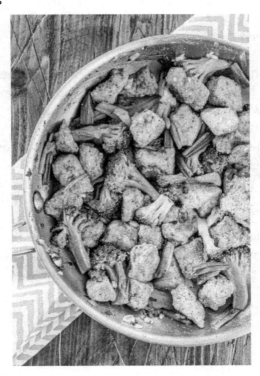

Tofu with Peas

Servings: 5
Preparation Time: 15 minutes
Cooking Time: 20 minutes

Ingredients:

- 2 tablespoons olive oil, divided
- 1 (16-ounce) package extra-firm tofu, drained, pressed and cubed
- 1 cup yellow onion, chopped
- 1 tablespoon fresh ginger, minced
- 2 garlic cloves, minced
- 1 tomato, chopped finely
- 2 cups frozen peas, thawed
- ¼ cup water
- 2 tablespoons fresh cilantro, chopped

Instructions:

1. In a non-stick wok, heat 1 tablespoon of the oil over medium-high heat and cook the tofu for about 4-5 minutes or until browned completely, stirring occasionally.
2. Transfer the tofu into a bowl.
3. In the same wok, heat the remaining oil over medium heat and sauté the onion for about 3-4 minutes.
4. Add the ginger and garlic and sauté for about 1 minute.
5. Add the tomatoes and cook for about 4-5 minutes, crushing with the back of a spoon.
6. Stir in the peas and broth and cook for about 2-3 minutes.
7. Stir in the tofu and cook for about 1-2 minutes.
8. Serve hot with the garnishing of cilantro.

Nutritional Information per Serving:

Calories: 291
Fat: 11.8g
Carbohydrates: 20g
Fiber: 10g
Sugar: 9g
Protein: 19g
Sodium: 732mg

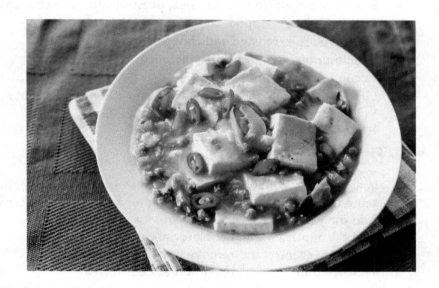

Tofu with Brussels Sprout

Servings: 3
Preparation Time: 15 minutes
Cooking Time: 15 minutes

Ingredients:

- 1 ½ tablespoons olive oil, divided
- 8 ounces extra-firm tofu, drained, pressed and cut into slices
- 2 garlic cloves, chopped
- 1/3 cup pecans, toasted and chopped
- 1 tablespoon unsweetened applesauce
- ¼ cup fresh cilantro, chopped
- ½ pound Brussels sprouts, trimmed and cut into wide ribbons
- ¾ pound mixed bell peppers, seeded and sliced

Instructions:

1. In a wok, heat ½ tablespoon of the oil over medium heat and sauté the tofu and for about 6-7 minutes or until golden brown.
2. Add the garlic and pecans and sauté for about 1 minute.
3. Add the applesauce and cook for about 2 minutes.
4. Stir in the cilantro and remove from heat.
5. Transfer tofu into a plate and set aside
6. In the same wok, heat the remaining oil over medium-high heat and cook the Brussels sprouts and bell peppers for about 5 minutes.
7. Stir in the tofu and remove from the heat.
8. Serve immediately.

Nutritional Information per Serving:

Calories: 238
Fat: 16g
Carbohydrates: 13g
Fiber: 4.8g
Sugar: 4.5g
Protein: 11.8g
Sodium: 26mg

Tofu with Veggies

Servings: 4
Preparation Time: 20 minutes
Cooking Time: 45 minutes

Ingredients:

- 1 (14-ounce) package extra firm tofu, pressed, drained and cut into small cubes
- 2 tablespoons sesame oil, divided
- 4 tablespoons low-sodium soy sauce
- 3 tablespoons maple syrup
- 2 tablespoons peanut butter
- 2 tablespoons fresh lime juice
- 1-2 teaspoons chili garlic sauce
- 1-pound green beans, trimmed
- 2-3 small red bell peppers, seeded and cubed
- 2 scallion greens, chopped

Instructions:

1. Preheat your oven to 400 degrees F.
2. Line a baking sheet with parchment paper.
3. Arrange the tofu cubes onto the prepared baking sheet in a single layer.
4. Bake for approximately 25-30 minutes.
5. Meanwhile, in a small bowl, add 1 tablespoon of the sesame oil, soy sauce, maple syrup, peanut butter, lime juice, and chili garlic sauce and beat until well combined. Set aside.
6. Remove from the oven and place the tofu cubes into the bowl of sauce.
7. Stir the mixture well and set aside for about 10 minutes, stirring occasionally.
8. With a slotted spoon, remove the tofu cubes from bowl, reserving the sauce.
9. Heat a large cast-iron wok over medium heat and cook the tofu cubes for about 5 minutes, stirring occasionally.

10. With a slotted spoon, transfer the tofu cubes onto a plate. Set aside.
11. In the same wok, add the remaining sesame oil, green beans, bell peppers and 2-3 tablespoons of reserved sauce and cook, covered for about 4-5 minutes.
12. Adjust the heat to medium-high, and stir in the cooked tofu remaining reserved sauce.
13. Cook for about 1-2 minutes, stirring frequently.
14. Stir in the scallion greens and serve hot.

Nutritional Information per Serving:

Calories: 320
Fat: 19g
Carbohydrates: 22g
Fiber: 6g
Sugar: 10g
Protein: 17.2g
Sodium: 129mg

Tofu & Mushroom Curry

Servings: 4
Preparation Time: 20 minutes
Cooking Time: 25 minutes

Ingredients:

For Tofu:

- 16 ounces extra-firm tofu, pressed, drained and cut into ½-inch cubes
- 1 garlic clove, minced
- 3 tablespoons balsamic vinegar
- 3 tablespoons low-sodium soy sauce
- 3 tablespoons arrowroot starch
- 2 tablespoons sesame oil
- 1 tablespoon Erythritol
- 1 teaspoon red pepper flakes
- 2 tablespoons coconut oil

For Curry:

- ¼ cup water
- 1 small yellow onion, minced
- 3 large garlic cloves, minced
- 1 teaspoon fresh ginger, grated
- 2 cups fresh mushrooms, sliced
- 3 tablespoons red curry paste
- 13 ounces light coconut milk
- 1 tablespoon low-sodium soy sauce
- 2 tablespoons fresh lime juice
- 1 teaspoon lime zest, grated
- 8 fresh basil leaves, chopped

Instructions:

1. For tofu: in a resealable bag, place all ingredients.

2. Seal the bag and shake to coat well.
3. Refrigerate to marinate for 2-4 hours.
4. In a large wok, melt the coconut oil over medium heat and stir fry the tofu cubes for about 4-5 minutes or until golden brown completely.
5. With a slotted spoon, transfer the tofu cubes into a bowl.
6. For curry: in a large pan, add the water over medium heat and ring to a simmer.
7. Add the minced onion, garlic and ginger and cook for about 5 minutes.
8. Add the mushrooms and curry paste and stir to combine well.
9. Stir in the remaining ingredients except for basil and simmer for about 10 minutes.
10. Stir in the tofu and simmer for about 5 minutes.
11. Garnish with basil and serve.

Nutritional Information per Serving:

Calories: 399
Fat: 25g
Carbohydrates: 15g
Fiber: 1.6g
Sugar: 4.1g
Protein: 14.4g
Sodium: 940mg

Tofu & Veggies Curry

Servings: 5
Preparation Time: 20 minutes
Cooking Time: 30 minutes

Ingredients:

- 1 (16-ounce) block firm tofu, drained, pressed and cut into ½-inch cubes
- 2 tablespoons coconut oil
- 1 medium yellow onion, chopped
- 1½ tablespoons fresh ginger, minced
- 2 garlic cloves, minced
- 1 tablespoon curry powder
- Salt and ground black pepper, as required
- 1 cup fresh mushrooms, sliced
- 1 cup carrots, peeled and sliced
- 1 (14-ounce) can unsweetened low-fat coconut milk
- ½ cup low-sodium vegetable broth
- 2 teaspoons Erythritol
- 10 ounces cauliflower florets
- 1 tablespoon fresh lime juice
- ¼ cup fresh basil leaves, sliced thinly

Instructions:

1. In a Dutch oven, heat the oil over medium heat and sauté the onion, ginger and garlic for about 5 minutes.
2. Stir in the curry powder, salt and black pepper and cook for about 2 minutes, stirring occasionally.
3. Add the mushrooms and carrot and cook for about 4-5 minutes.
4. Stir in the coconut milk, broth and brown sugar and bring to a boil.
5. Add the tofu and cauliflower and simmer for about 12-15 minutes, stirring occasionally.
6. Stir in the lime juice and remove from the heat.
7. Serve hot.

Nutritional Information per Serving:

Calories: 330
Fat: 16g
Carbohydrates: 18g
Fiber: 6g
Sugar: 8g
Protein: 17.2g
Sodium: 129mg

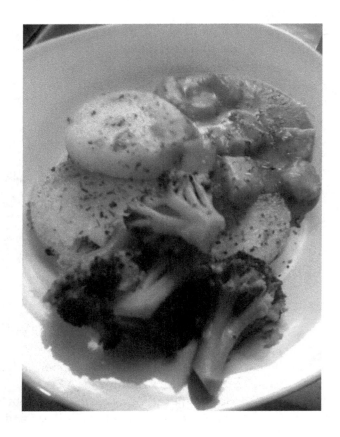

Tempeh with Bell Peppers

Servings: 3
Preparation Time: 15 minutes
Cooking Time: 15 minutes

Ingredients:

- 2 tablespoons balsamic vinegar
- 2 tablespoons low-sodium soy sauce
- 2 tablespoons tomato sauce
- 1 teaspoon maple syrup
- ½ teaspoon garlic powder
- 1/8 teaspoon red pepper flakes, crushed
- 1 tablespoon vegetable oil
- 8 ounces tempeh, cut into cubes
- 1 medium onion, chopped
- 2 large green bell peppers, seeded and chopped

Instructions:

1. In a small bowl, add the vinegar, soy sauce, tomato sauce, maple syrup, garlic powder and red pepper flakes and beat until well combined. Set aside.
2. Heat 1 tablespoon of oil in a large wok over medium heat and cook the tempeh about 2-3 minutes per side.
3. Add the onion and bell peppers and heat for about 2-3 minutes.
4. Stir in the sauce mixture and cook for about 3-5 minutes, stirring frequently.
5. Serve hot.

Nutritional Information per Serving:

Calories: 291
Fat: 11.9g
Carbohydrates: 23g
Fiber: 10g
Sugar: 10g
Protein: 19g
Sodium: 732mg

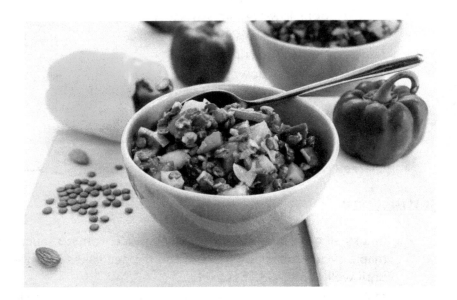

Tempeh with Brussel Sprout & Kale

Servings: 3
Preparation Time: 15 minutes
Cooking Time: 17 minutes

Ingredients:

- 2 tablespoons olive oil
- 1/3 cup red onion, chopped finely
- 1 ½ cups tempeh, cubed
- 2 cups Brussels sprout, quartered
- 2 garlic cloves, minced
- ½ teaspoon ground cumin
- ½ teaspoon garlic powder
- Salt and ground black pepper, as required
- 2 cups fresh kale, tough ribs removed and chopped

Instructions:

1. Heat the oil in a wok over medium-high heat and sauté the onion for about 4-5 minutes.
2. Add in remaining ingredients except for kale and cook for about 6-7 minutes, stirring occasionally.
3. Add kale and cook for about 5 minutes, stirring twice.
4. Serve hot.

Nutritional Information per Serving:

Calories: 291
Fat: 18.8g
Carbohydrates: 18g
Fiber: 3.3g
Sugar: 2g
Protein: 18.g
Sodium: 86mg

Tempeh with Veggies

Servings: 3
Preparation Time: 15 minutes
Cooking Time: 17 minutes

Ingredients:

For Sauce:

- 3 tablespoons tahini
- 2 tablespoons low-sodium soy sauce
- 1 tablespoon sesame oil
- 1 tablespoon chili-garlic sauce
- 1 tablespoon maple syrup

For tempeh & Veggies:

- 3 tablespoons olive oil, divided
- 8 ounces tempeh, cut into 1x2-inch rectangular strips
- 8 ounces fresh button mushrooms, sliced thinly
- 8 ounces fresh spinach
- 1 tablespoon fresh ginger, minced
- 1 tablespoon garlic, minced

Instructions:

1. For sauce: in a bowl, add all ingredients and beat until well combined.
2. In a large wok, heat the oil over medium-high heat and cook the tempeh for about 4-5 minutes or until browned.
3. With a slotted spoon, transfer the tempeh into a bowl and set aside.
4. In the same wok, heat the remaining oil over medium-high heat and cook the mushrooms for about 6-7 minutes, stirring frequently.
5. With a slotted spoon, transfer the mushrooms into a bowl and set aside.

6. In the same wok, add the spinach, ginger and garlic and cook for about 2-3 minutes.
7. Stir in the cooked tempeh, mushrooms and sauce and cook for about 1-2 minutes, stirring continuously.
8. Serve hot.

Nutritional Information per Serving:

Calories: 341
Fat: 26.5g
Carbohydrates: 15g
Fiber: 2.9g
Sugar: 4.8g
Protein: 16.5g
Sodium: 100mg

CPSIA information can be obtained
at www.ICGtesting.com
Printed in the USA
BVHW092133090621
609092BV00002B/374